Gua-Sh

The Natural Massage and Self Treatment Guide to Maintain a Healthy Face and Skin

Melk Joe

Table of Contents

Introduction

Gua-sha is a part of the Traditional Chinese Medication (TCM). It is also known as "scraping", "spooning", or "coining". It is used professionally as an instrument to scrape people's pores and skin, it is said to have a therapeutic advantage. The procedure of this particular medication has a French name called *tribo-effleurage*. Gua-sha is an all-natural option therapy that involves scraping your skin layer with a therapeutic massage tool to boost your blood circulation. This ancient Chinese curing technique provides a unique method for better health and also deals with issues like chronic pain.

In Gua-sha, a technician scrapes your skin layer with brief or long strokes to stimulate microcirculation of the smooth cells, which increases blood circulation; they make these strokes with a smooth-edged device known as a *Gua-therapeutic massage tool*, the specialist applies massage essential oil to your skin layer, and then uses the tool to scrape your skin layer in a downward movement frequently. Gua-sha is supposed to handle stagnant energy called *chi*, professionals believe that this *"chi"* is responsible for swellings in any part of the body. Swelling is the reason behind several conditions associated with chronic pain. Massaging the skin's surface is considered to help split up this energy, reduce irritation and promote recovery.

Gua-sha is usually performed on the back, buttocks, neck, hands and legs. A mild version of it is even applied to the facial skin as a cosmetic technique. Your specialist may apply moderate pressure and then steadily increase strength to regulate how much pressure you are designed for.

Chapter 1

What is Face Gua Sha?

Face Gua-Sha is a well-known scraping massage technique made by Traditional Chinese Medicine. It started as a remedy done exclusively on your own body to boost blood circulation, move lymphatic stagnation, and releases muscle tension. After a while, a much gentler version was designed for the facial skin, that involves a light gliding motion tone that lifts and smooths your skin layer. Tools of assorted shapes made of crystal (*such as the jade or rose quartz*) are found in mixture with light pressure in an upward and downward movement.

The target is to de-puff the facial skin by facilitating lymphatic drainage into the neck and bring fresh blood & nutrients to your skin layer for a healthy glow. As you softly scrape your skin layer, micro-circulation is usually improved which carries oxygenated bloodstream towards the dermal layers clearing congestion, stimulating cell renewal and brightening your appearance. This hurry of blood brings nutrients that produces cell regeneration and tissues repair which is far more productive and incredibly helpful if you're dealing with acne or want to eliminate acne scarring.

Overall, it's an amazingly easy addition to your early morning or evening epidermis routine that demands 5 minutes and will give you noticeable lift and shine every time.

Gua-Sha Tools

Long ago, Gua-Sha scraping tools were made of things such as: bones and even cow horns. I was once told that cow horns are excellent conductors of vigour, as cows use their horns to communicate. I have no idea of how true the myth is, although I'd want to trust the idea of telepathic cows. However, it is wise that crystals are used today because they're also considered to emit energy.

Advantages of Gua-sha

Cosmetic Gua-Sha movement is a lymphatic liquid that gets built-up in the facial skin, which bears away poisons that may contribute to acne and boring irritated skin.

Gua-Sha does the following:

- Shades the muscles from the facial skin that may assist with sagging skin.

- Companies and hydrates your skin layer.

- Relaxes muscle stress in the facial skin, increasing full body stress alleviation (puts the body in a parasympathetic condition, which is wonderful for those who have trouble drifting off to sleep).

- Boosts blood flow & circulation.

- Moves stagnant bloodstream that plays a component role in dark circles & under-eye bags.

- Helps your skin layer overcome blemishes & acne scars.

- Prevents lines and wrinkles and helps erase existing lines

- De-puffs and slims the facial skin.

- Instantly lifts and plumps your skin layer.

- Allows serums to penetrate deeper post-treatment.

- Soothes throat pain & headache because of tight

muscle or fascia.

How to Perform Gua-sha at home

If you wish to begin with the throat/jaw and then work your path up, that means you beginning lymphatic drainage at the least expensive stage, that way when you get up to your forehead and vision area, the liquid and poisons have someplace to drain into as being a funnel.

Additionally, you intend to use very light pressure; if your skin layer begins to get very red, it is to company rather than concentrating on the lymph. Lymph needs light-weight because your lymphatic vessels are close to the top, your tools ought to be angled at about 15-20, almost smooth to your skin layer in order to ensure that you're not stabbing yourself and experience the soft pull that plays a component in the lifting impact.

Always scrape towards outer sides from the facial skin and sweep down from the guts when you're doing all of your neck, meaning your lymph drains appropriately in to the nodes above your collarbone.

How Important is the Lymphatic System?

Do you realize your lymphatic system is doubly significant as your circulatory system? While your circulatory system has your center to pump as well as clean your bloodstream automatically, your lymph doesn't have any built-in pump whatsoever. The lymph just goes on through exercise, massage therapy and diet which is why it's straightforward to get supported by this modern lifestyle.

The lymphatic system was not fully understood under the western culture until significantly less than 2 decades ago - yet ancient systems of medicine such as TCM or Ayurveda view is probably the first places to consider stagnation whenever you're ill. The AMA historically ignores lymph stagnation as causes of disease, whereas other countries such as Germany use specific Lymphatic Drainage techniques as an end to fibrocystic breast disease, allergies, persistent sinusitis, arthritis, eczema, coronary disease and more.

An indicator that your lymphatic system is sluggish is:

- If your body were a residence, think about your blood as the tap and your lymph as the drains. As I said, your bloodstream is always pumping, meaning your valves are continually operating. The problem is that they run straight into the region that it isn't nonetheless assured to visit. When sending particles from your bloodstream that are too large to be removed from your liver organ, kidneys, or epidermis, it goes straight into your lymphatic vessels. So when those "drains" aren't moving steadily, stagnation and disease occur.

The most typical causes of poor lymphatic circulation are:

- **Stress** - The chemistry of stress is degenerative and lymph-congesting in character. Overwork and insufficient rest periods bargain your lymph, digestion of food, and liver organ Qi.

- **Digestive Imbalances** - Irritation from the intestinal villi credited to inflammatory foods and poor digestion congests us because almost all your lymph surrounds the gut via "Gut Associated

Lymph Tissue" (GALT). Check out what I said later in this book about 11 uncommon (yet straightforward) methods to increase your digestion. To obtain additional in-depth solutions, I've clarified the four main causes of poor digestion and just how to address most of them.

- **Deficiencies** - Nutrient deficiencies especially iodine impact the lymph. Iodine really helps to mitigate the results of the harmful environment (hello pesticide-sprayed world!) and supports the lymph at a mobile level. Check what I wrote on the advantages of seaweed.

- **Emotions/Religion** - Shame, blocked circulation of pleasure in life, depression, repressed emotions.

- **Inactivity** - Since I explained that this lymph doesn't have any pump and that it depends on you to work. An inactive lifestyle/working a table job seriously compromises lymphatic flow.

- **Diet** - Foods can either help or avoid the blast of lymph. Most unfortunately prepared/packaged, processed sugars (corn syrup), white flour affects the lymph.

Face Gua-Sha is one small section of the lymphatic puzzle, nonetheless it helps to get things moving, especially if you have chronic issues with mucus build-up within your sinuses.

Actions you may take to improve lymphatic blood flow include:

- Take strolls everyday especially after meals (might just be for ten minutes).

- Eat the white section of the orange! (click that to know more about my post on this).

- Consume red-stainned foods (pure cranberry juice, blueberries, and raspberries).

- Reduce how often you sit back each day each. Give dry-brushing a rebound for just a few minutes, several times a day.

Chapter 2

Beauty Restored - The Advantages of Face Gua-Sha

Transform your tone with these facial massage therapy techniques. You are able to tell a whole lot about someone by merely looking at their face, not merely the manifestation of their pulling or the immediate feel. But health and fitness will also be written on your face, and that's because, according to Chinese medication, your beauty is definitely an external representation of the internal health.

So our beauty routines are definite improvements to your overall health. Our creator and resident physician, Katie, has captured the substance of a lot of long time Chinese wisdom into some powerful one-minute rituals. Quick and straightforward to accomplish, they are able to fit neatly into our modern lives, offering a transformative approach to health and fitness, subsequently providing you with a healthy, glowing and radiant tone.

Recreate Your Beauty

We're likely to demonstrate three iconic Chinese approaches for improving your appearance, we've processed them and this implies that they may be done in minutes. And that means a minute to each.

They may be *Àn-fa* (*press-hold*) *Gua-Sha* (*press stroke*) and *Acupressure* (*press-turn*).

It has been within the Chinese facial massage therapy for several years and revered due to its restorative and chilling properties.

Our studies showed that 82% of women found an instantaneous and positive impact after just one single minute use.

- **Àn-fa**

In this technique, you will need to press and support the jade Beauty RestorerTM over your face; press-holding the jade may reduce swelling and increase lymphatic drainage.

You place take the sweetness RestorerTM around the

eyes to ease fatigue, alleviate eyesight bags, puffy eye, or twitching eyes muscles. You can also utilize the jade tool over any region to help ease stress-related symptoms such as for example headaches, flushing, epidermis circumstances, and throbbing temples.

- **Gua-Sha**

Gua-Sha is an easy press and heart stroke technique along the curves of your face, as shown. This beauty treatment continues to be used across Asia for many years. It is renown for it's unique capacity to increase blood circulation under your skin layer, bringing in nourishment and improve collagen.

So, instead of applying a cream or serum to improve your skin layer from the surface, you're activating your body to nourish your skin layer in an even more profound and meaningful way. This self-massage technique has shown in studies to boost circulation by 100%. It stimulates the dermis to assist collagen creation, manipulating parts of stress to relax cosmetic muscles, exponentially raises bloodstream and lymphatic movement. All this leads to a brighter, healthier and more radiant tone.

- **Acupressure**

Activating acupressure factor on your face is an excellent way to assist your organs internally. Chinese medication recognizes that cosmetic beauty is usually from your organs this way – i.e it reveals your overall health.

Chapter 3

Gua-Sha Materials: Comprehensive

Check out the list below and you will see the very best materials to consider:

1.   Bian Stone

Bian stones are thought to be the very best tools for Gua-sha because they probably have the most ultrasonic pulses and the very best collection of frequency, using Bian stones for therapy is centuries old. In the "Nei Jing," a historical Chinese Medical publication, it lists "acupuncture, moxibustion, natural medication, Qigong and Bian rock therapy" as the five primary medical ways of the "Yellow Emperor," a deity in Chinese religious beliefs. What's impressive is that Bian rock therapy predates acupuncture.

If you want to do Gua-Sha the authentic way, use Bian rocks.

2.   Jade

Jade is our second best pick for Gua-sha devices. It is known to possess qi energy that's nearly the qi vigour of your body. Therefore, it is really ideal for healing treatments. In the olden times, barefoot doctors in China cannot afford traditional Gua-sha tools, so they got scraps from jade carvers and used them as Gua-sha tools. Today, jade is still widely used as a result of it's healing technique.

3.   Buffalo Horn

Genuine Bian rocks are gotten from the city of Sibin in China. If you can't get Bian rocks to use, Buffalo horn is another excellent option.

In Chinese medicine, a buffalo horn includes a chilly property and an acrid/salty flavor. The acridity enhances qi and blood circulation, nourishes, and moistens. The saltiness alternatively relaxes, tightness and softens hardness. Finally, the coldness dispels warmth and eliminates poisons in the body.

While American buffalo are from your endangered list, in the event that you worry about where buffalo horns are gotten from, obtain jade, natural stone or steel instead.

4.   Stainless Steel

Medical-grade stainless tools certainly are a favorite choice for DASCM (Device Assisted Soft Cells Mobilization) and so are only a modern development of Gua-Sha. If you want newer materials, you should consider Stainless and even Titanium implements.

5.   Rose Quartz

Rose quartz is known to open up the guts chakra and reduce pressure in the guts. It is a pleasant stone that can be found in a delicate red colorization.

Just like a Gua-Sha tool, it is really smooth and has an excellent weight. Others though believe that it is hard to carry and pick the buffalo horn or bian rock. Any object - as being a coin, a spoon or a cover - can be employed for Gua-Sha. Acquiring the best material, though, makes the entire experience convenient and with techniques, it becomes even more memorable as you utilize tools that becomes special to you.

Like that of a historical recovery, you'll manage your stress and diseases in more natural ways instead of relying on pharmaceuticals or higher vices that only bring short-term alleviation.

Gua-Sha Jade Stone

Gua-Sha for the facial skin and neck is known as the Eastern Botox or Eastern Facelift for grounds. This Traditional Chinese Medication treatment, when placed on the facial skin gets the next results:

- ✓ Companies up your sagging face muscles.

- ✓ Smoothens your skin layer and reduces the lines and wrinkles on your face.

- ✓ Improves dark circles and eyebags beneath the eye (the sort you get from advancing generation)

- ✓ Lightens age places and other epidermis discolorations.

- ✓ Your tone gets rosier and more radiant.

- ✓ Helps remove acne, rosacea and additional epidermis diseases on your face.

How to use:

Our Rose Quartz Gua-Sha tools include a printed beginner's guide to obtain the most from it at home.

Konjac Face Sponge - Pure

Perfect for everyone, a 100% Pure Konjac Sponge deeply cleanses, eliminates blackheads and gently exfoliates your skin layer. The initial online like framework from the veggie fibers really helps to stimulate blood flow and promote epidermis cell renewal.

How to use:

Before use, wash the sponge thoroughly. We recommend plunging it in normal water and squeezing it often. If the sponge is dry, allow it to fully absorb water before putting it against your skin layer.

Softly massage the facial skin and body in a circular motion round to exfoliate dead skin cells and cleanse deeply. The massage will stimulate exhausted epidermis & encourage epidermis renewal. Soap or cleansing solution could be placed into the sponge if desired but it isn't essential.

Your sponge should last almost a year, but once it begins to look tired or breakdown. Please replace it. The better treatment you consider of the sponge, the longer it'll last.

Konjac Face Sponge - Bamboo Charcoal

Filled with nutrient-rich triggered carbon, the Konjac Sponge with Bamboo Charcoal deeply cleans pores to eliminate blackheads and dirt and grime while absorbing extra oils and toxins. An all-natural antioxidant, it kills persistent acne-causing bacteria and is a natural efficient treatment of acne.

How to use:

Before use, wash the sponge thoroughly. We recommend plunging it in normal water and squeezing it often. If the sponge is dry, allow it to fully absorb water before putting it against your skin layer

Lightly massage the facial skin and body in a circular motion round, to exfoliate dead skin cells, and cleanse deeply. The massage will stimulate exhausted epidermis & encourage epidermis renewal. Soap or cleansing solution could be placed into the sponge if desired but isn't essential.

Your sponge should last almost a year, but once it begins

to look tired or breakdown. Please replace it. The better treatment you consider of the sponge, the longer it'll last.

Konjac Face Sponge - Green Tea Herb

Green tea extract herb is naturally filled with antioxidants which have a cell-protecting function, they perform a considerable antioxidant impact that protects your skin layer from the damaging effect of free radicals. This natural component includes a softening and plumping influence on boosting elasticity and refreshing your skin's appearance, which would work for those who desire to protect their skin from aging.

How to use:

Before use, wash the sponge thoroughly. We recommend plunging it in normal water and squeezing it often. If the sponge is dry, allow it to fully absorb water before putting it against your skin layer.

Softly massage the facial skin and body in a circular motion round to exfoliate dead skin cells and cleanse deeply. The massage will stimulate exhausted epidermis & encourage epidermis renewal. Soap or cleansing solution could be placed into the sponge if desired but it isn't essential.

Your sponge should last almost a year, but once it begins to look tired or breakdown. Please replace it. The better treatment you consider of the sponge, the longer it'll last.

Konjac Face Sponge - Folks from France Pink Clay

An ideal Konjac Sponge for all the exceptional extremes from the components of air-con, excess sun exposure, and central heating. Pure French Red Clay softly purifies even the most delicate epidermis and includes a softening and plumping effect on boosting elasticity and refreshes your skin's appearance.

How to use:

Before use, wash the sponge thoroughly. We recommend plunging it in normal water and squeezing it often. If the sponge is dry, allow it to fully absorb water before putting it against your skin layer.

Softly massage the facial skin and body in a circular

motion round to exfoliate dead skin cells and cleanse deeply. The massage will stimulate exhausted epidermis & encourage epidermis renewal. Soap or cleansing solution could be placed into the sponge if desired but it isn't essential.

Your sponge should last almost a year, but once it begins to look tired or breakdown. Please replace it. The better treatment you consider of the sponge, the longer it'll last.

Konjac Face Sponge - Lavender

Lavender can be an all-natural relaxant and detoxifier with impressive recovery capabilities. This beautiful blossom has strong skills to relax and reduce stress and anxious tension, rendering it perfect for soothing skin treatment.

How to use:

Before use, wash the sponge thoroughly. We recommend plunging it in normal water and squeezing it often. If the sponge is dry, allow it to fully absorb water before putting it against your skin layer.

Softly massage the facial skin and body in a circular

motion round to exfoliate dead skin cells and cleanse deeply. The massage will stimulate exhausted epidermis & encourage epidermis renewal. Soap or cleansing solution could be placed into the sponge if desired but it isn't essential.

Your sponge should last almost a year, but once it begins to look tired or breakdown. Please replace it. The better treatment you consider of the sponge, the longer it'll last.

Chapter 4

What are the Advantages of Gua-Sha?

Gua-sha may reduce swelling, so it's often used to deal with illnesses that cause chronic pain, such as arthritis and fibromyalgia, as well as those that bring about muscle and joint pain.

Gua-sha may possibly relieve symptoms of other conditions like:

1. Hepatitis B

Hepatitis B is a viral contamination that triggers liver inflammation, liver harm and liver scarring. Research has proven that Gua-sha may reduce persistent liver inflammation.

A trusted research study followed up a man with high liver enzymes, a sign of liver irritation. He was offered Gua-sha medication, and after 48 hours of treatment, he experienced a reduction in his liver enzymes. However, some experts also believe that Gua-sha can aid against liver swelling, thus decreasing the likelihood of liver harm. More research is underway.

2. Migraine headaches

Should your migraine persist after you've taken several "over-the-counter medications", Gua-sha might help. A report from a reliable source asserts that a 72-year-old female dealing with chronic headaches received Gua-sha a lot more in 2 weeks, and her migraines were relieved during this time period, suggesting that this ancient curing technique could be an efficient fix for problems.

3. Breast engorgement

Breast engorgement is a problem experienced by many breastfeeding women i.e. when the chest is overfilled with dairy, this usually occurs in the first weeks of breastfeeding. The mother's breast becomes inflamed and painful, rendering it difficult for babies to latch. However, this is usually a short-term condition.

Study asserts that women receive Gua-sha from the very next day after expecting until departing a healthcare facility. A healthcare facility adopted the gua-sha medication on women in the weeks after expecting, and they found that most of them experienced relief from engorgement i.e breasts fullness and pain, this thus allowed breastfeeding to become easier for them.

4. Neck pain

Also, the Gua-sha technique is an effective fix for chronic throat pain. To consider the potency of the therapy, 48 research participants were placed into two groups. One group was offered gua-sha, while the other group used a thermal heat pad to deal with the throat pain. After a week, people who received gua-sha reported less pain compared to the group that didn't receive gua-sha.

5. Tourette syndrome

The symptoms of Tourette include involuntary motions such as face tics, neck clearing and vocal outbursts associated with a person. Gua-sha in conjunction with various other therapies may help to reduce symptoms of Tourette in the person being analysed.

The analysis involved a 33-year-old male who had Tourette syndrome at age 9, he received acupuncture, natural herbs, gua-sha and altered his lifestyle, his symptoms relieved by 70 percent. Despite him testing positive, further research is essential.

6. Premenopausal syndrome

Pre-menopausal occurs in women near menopause. Symptoms include:

- Insomnia.

- Irregular periods.

- Anxiety.

- Fatigue.

- Hot flashes

Studies, however, has shown that gua-sha may reduce premenopausal symptoms in a few women. The analysis examined 80 women with premenopausal symptoms. The procedure group received 15 tiny gua-sha treatments once weekly, as well as standard therapy for eight weeks. *The control group only received regular therapy.*

Upon completion of the analysis, the involvement group reported an increased reduction of symptoms such as insomnia, anxiety, exhaustion, headaches and hot flashes compared to the control group.

Experts believe gua-sha therapy may be considered a safe and effective treatment for these symptoms.

Does Gua-sha have Side Effects?

As an all-natural healing treatment, gua-sha is safe. It's not reported to be unpleasant, however the procedure may change the looks of your skin layer since it entails massaging or scraping epidermis, having a massage therapy tool, tiny arteries referred to as capillaries near the surface of your skin layer may burst, this might lead to epidermis bruising and small loss of blood. Bruising usually disappears in a few days.

A lot of people also experience short-term indentation of their epidermis after a gua-sha treatment.

The following are the three necessary precautions to be taken:

- If any bleeding occurs, there are chances of transferring blood-borne illnesses with gua-sha therapy, so technicians must disinfect their tools after each person.

- Avoid this technique if you've undergone any surgery in the last six weeks.

Individuals who are taking bloodstream thinners or have clotting disorders aren't suitable applicants for gua-sha.

Chapter 5

Uses of Gua-sha

Listed here are various ways of gua-sha meditation technique:

- Gua-sha is generally used to ease muscle and joint pain. Complications from the muscles and bone tissue are referred to as musculoskeletal disorders, several examples include back pain, tendon stress and carpal tunnel symptoms.

- Practitioners declare that gua-sha also offers the benefit of fighting disease and reduce amount of irritation. Sometimes, gua-sha is useful to look after a chill, fever or problems with the lungs.

- Small injuries to the body, just like the bruises due to gua-sha, are now and again referred to as micro-trauma. These produce a reply in the body that might help seperate scar tissue formation. Micro-trauma also can help with fibrosis, which can be an accumulation of an excessive amount of connective tissue whenever your body heals.

- Physiotherapists might use IASTM on connective cells that aren't wanting to move bones, this problem could be credited to repetitive stress damage or another condition. Gua-sha could be used alongside other treatments, such as extending and conditioning exercises.

Great Things about Gua-Sha

Researchers have completed small studies on another sets of individuals to learn if gua-sha works. They are:

- Women near menopause.

- People using the guitar neck, to help to reduce pain from computer use.

- Male weightlifters: To aid recovery after training.

- Old adults with back pain.

- Women found with pre-menopausal symptoms such as perspiration, insomnia and headaches reported that these symptoms were reduced after gua-sha.

A 2014 study found that gua-sha improved the amount of

motion and reduce pain in individuals who used personal computers frequently. Also, another research in 2017 revealed that weightlifters who have had gua-sha therapy found it better to lift weight after treatment.

Old adults with back pain were treated with either gua-sha or a hot pack, both treatments relieved symptoms similarly well. However, the effects of gua-sha lasted a lot longer. A week after, those that had received gua-sha treatment reported greater versatility and less back pain compared to the other group.

Adverse Effects and Risk

Gua-sha often burst tiny arteries near the surface of your skin layer called the capillaries. It generates a distinctive red or crimson bruise, referred to as "sha". The injuries usually last for a few days or weeks and may be tender while healing. People might take an over-the-counter painkiller, such as Ibuprofen to aid the pain and reduce bloating. A person should protect the bruised region and become mindful not to bump it. (Applying a snowpack might help reduce swelling and simplicity in any pain).

Gua-sha professionals shouldn't break your skin layer through the procedure, but there are risks that could happen. A cut on the surface escalates the possibility of illness, so gua-sha specialists should sterilize their tools between treatments.

Gua-sha isn't for everybody, people who should not undergo the therapy includes the following:

- Those who have medical ailments on their skin or in their veins.

- Those who bleed very easily.

- Those who take medication to thin their blood.

- Those who have deep vein thrombosis.

- Those who have experienced contamination, tumor or wound that hasn't healed fully.

- Those who come with an implant, just like a pacemaker or internal defibrillator.

Is Gua-sha Painful?

Treatment isn't reported to be painful but gua-sha

deliberately causes bruising which can cause discomfort for a number of people, these bruises should heal in just a few days.

Gua-sha Tools and Technique

Equipment used in Gua-Sha

A handheld tool with curved edges is employed in gua-sha. Typically, a spoon or coin will be employed to scrape your skin layer, however, in modern practice, therapists use just a little hand-held tool with rounded edges.

Gua-sha tools have a tendency to end up being weighed to greatly help the specialist doing the duty to apply pressure.

Professionals of Traditional East Asian Medication see some materials as using power that may support recovery - these materials include Bian rock, jade and rose quartz. Medical quality stainless is often utilized for IASTM or when gua-sha is conducted in an infirmary. Professionals will apply gas to the spot of the body that is being treated, this allows the therapist to utilize the tool over the skin more efficiently. The gua-sha practitioner will press these devices in to the body with smooth and firm strokes in one path. If Gua-sha continues to be completed around the trunk or back from the legs, a person may need to lay face down on a massage therapy table.

Chapter 6

Gua-Sha: The DIY Beauty Tool for an inside-out Glow

Self-care and skincare may actually move together, Eva Ramirez explores the historic ritual of Gua-sha and just how it could promote medical health insurance and radiance from within.

Gua-sha (pronounced *gwa-sha*) is definitely an old self-care practice in traditional Chinese medicine. Whenever a tool, usually produced from jade, bone or horn, is scraped over the skin to redirect energy stream, using this method stagnant energy is divided, reducing irritation, increasing blood flow and stimulating the lymphatic system to promote healing in the body. It's an easy but demanding technique that has been in use for a very long time to take care of problems such as fever, muscle pain and pressure, swelling, chronic coughs, sinusitis and migraines.

Self-care is a center point of Chinese Medication, where it is really named Yang Sheng (healthy life).

Traditionally, Gua-sha was practiced in the home, as one of the numerous historical wellness customs, it became more popular under western culture. Much like cupping or acupressure, many acupuncturists and professionals offer Gua-sha massage therapy as a remedy in their centers. Like an athletic therapeutic massage, but having a prop, it is carried out with a medium to reduce pressure around a person's neck, legs and arms, honing in on whichever areas specifically needs attention. The friction from your repeated strokes leads to scary-looking bruising and inflammation that may last for some time after treatment.

Why Should We Make Dry Body Cleaning a Normal Habit?

Just what does this has to do with beauty and skincare? Well, a gentler version from the Gua-sha technique works just like a miracle when applied on the facial skin. In this case, you don't need to visit a therapist because everything, in regards to your skin care and wellbeing is being looked after through your regular everyday skincare.

Can a Reiki Face Heal Your Skin Layer?

All you have to do is get a Gua-sha tool in regards to a minute every day application to see instant results and long-term benefits. Studies also show that everyday ritual enhances microcirculation by up to 100%, it reduces wrinkles, rejuvenates, tones and smoothen skin, boosts collagen, combats pigmentation, dark circles and puffy eyes, defines jawlines as well as decongests the sinuses.

It's literally like rubbing your path to healthy and glowing skin, because it primarily works through from within and to the surface, you'll also notice a release of tension and relaxing of facial muscles in the event that you clench your jaw at night. It is a sensible way to ease any soreness any day. In the event that you often get eye twitches from insomnia or stress, holding the Gua-sha over your eyes with gentle pressure may also support, relieve and relax the muscles.

To be certain you're using the proper tools for the task,

it's easier to get yourself a gua-sha made of jade. Aside from looking beautiful on your own dresser, this green rock is revered due to its air-con properties, steering clear of anything produced from bone and horn for apparent factors. It is also sensible to avoid cheaper alternatives that may be created from acrylic or additional artificial chemicals that may irritate your skin layer. Applying facial oil before massaging might help the stone to glide easily while moisturizing your skin layer too.

Katie Brindle is a Chinese medicine specialist and the creator of Hayo'u, an all-natural medical health insurance and skincare brand situated in the U.K. Hayo'u makes the self-treatment element of Chinese medication accessible and approachable with simple daily rituals and useful techniques. They offer the equipment such as their Gua-sha, which is usually carved from traditional Xiuyan Jade and carries a velvet pouch (ideal for traveling) as well as short easy-to-follow videos in order to perfect the ritual at home.

Weather practice may be the initial thing to do like an early morning ritual or as an evening wind-down to remove the day's stress from your face, this mindful beauty practice is usually meditative and relaxing.

Chapter 7

How to Perform Gua-sha on a Face in 11 Simple Steps

Once I notice it's likely you've had a Gua-Sha for your face and throat, I'd be amazed. I've been a lover of the historical treatment but didn't recognize that there's a face version.

Great things about Face Gua-Sha

Gua-Sha for the facial skin and neck, is known as the Eastern Botox (or Eastern Facelift). This traditional Chinese Medication treatment when placed on the facial skin does the following:

- Supports your sagging facial muscles.

- Smoothens your skin layer and reduces the lines and wrinkles on your face.

- Improves dark circles and eyebags beneath the eye (the sort you obtain from advancing generation).

- Lightens age and additional epidermis discolorations.

- Your tone gets rosier and more radiant.

- Helps remove acne, rosacea and other epidermis diseases on your face.

I've a first-hand experience with everything on the list apart from the last, and although I'm used to expecting great results because of my positive encounters with body Gua-Sha, I've been nonetheless amazed to start to see the improvements on my face.

I'd halted taking Glutathione and Grape Seed, but after a week or two of face Gua-Sha, my face includes a clearness and radiance that I'd just generally possess while on those supplements.

How it Works

As discussed above, Gua-Sha is identified as the age-old practice which involves the scraping movements all over the surface of one's body using a smooth-edged tool. It is really hard enough to boost petechial, reddish marks that typically transmit a Gua-Sha therapy program.

Gua-Sha Scraping

Face Gua-Sha is a lot much milder but has got the same scraping action along your skin layer, as your skin layer is scraped, the layers of your skin layer are activated and stagnant lymph that creates puffiness is usually relocated and cleared from the machine, poisons will also be released, creating a brighter appearance and finally, the massaging action relaxes anxious muscles that wrinkles provide.

Eastern Botox in 11 Steps

Many reminders for beginners:

- Don't utilize the same heavy pressure that you apply when scraping the body. If you want this to work, you should employ only light-weight. The facial skin is more delicate than other areas of the body.

- We are moving stagnant lymph from your face. We will drain this out via the proper and remaining lymphatic ducts. They are the areas among your collarbones.

- All our (light) scraping movements will be upwards. Remember; we are countering sagging, so we can not ever make any downward actions. The only exclusion may be the finished part if we do the dumping in the lymphatic ducts highlighted above.

Cosmetic Gua-Sha

Here are the general actions you are to take as a newbie:

- **Third Vision:** Heart stroke from the guts of the eyebrows or even more to your hairline. This region activates curing.

- **Lower forehead:** Sweep from your guts from the forehead above your eyebrows venturing out to your temples.

- **Under eyebrow:** Make use of the curve a part of your gua-sha tool to scrape the spot underneath your eyebrow and above your eye. Be mindful of the bone from the brow.

- **Under the attention:** Slowly and lightly stroke the spot where your vision bags typically show, start through the medial side of the nasal and rise to your temple. Imagine moving the stagnant lymph from the guts of your face up to the temple and entirely towards the hairline.

- **Cheek:** Do the same sweeping movement for the cheek area. Proceed in the medial side of the nasal, across your cheek or even more again to the guts of the ear.

- **Jaws:** Do the same for the jaws again, sweeping the lymph upwards to your ears.

- **Chin:** Sweep from the guts of your face, under your lower lip and to the earlobes.

- **Under chin:** Scrape from your soft field under your chin to underneath the ears.

- **Throat:** Finally, mild energy should be used to scrape from your own jaw and earlobes because of the center of the collarbone.

- **The very best sweep:** Collect all the lymph

you've moved aside from the facial skin and dump in your lymphatic drainage, sweep through the guts of the forehead right under your hairline, through your temple, your ears until you reach your throat and terminus area. Do it often for a clean sweep.

Chapter 8

How to Give Yourself the Best Gua-Sha Face at Home

What exactly does gua-sha do?

Gua-sha pre-dates acupuncture, the heart stroke design used to awaken the meridian lines (life force route) and to activate the body's natural curing abilities. For your skin layer, gua-sha stimulates collagen creation (power in cells), it sculpts and shades the facial skin, allowing irritation to drain and muscles to become free from pressure - permitting them to create their supportive paths properly. Also, it can help your skin get back to its most radiant condition as blood flow is usually increased, sending nutrition to areas that may have already been starved due to blockage.

Gua-Sha's impact is a lot more than epidermis deep as the meridian lines are enlivened. Organs like the belly, liver, spleen, center and kidneys also get a great advantage. Coping with gua-sha tools over the spot from the facial skin to the kidneys allows them to be used at an ideal capacity.

What are the Huge Benefits?

- Bears nutrient-rich and oxygenated bloodstream (food for the cells) to your skin layer and tissues.

- Drains lymph liquid (which is often loaded with poisons and spend) from your cells to become cleansed.

- Eliminates or considerably reduces wrinkles.

- Treats and aids in preventing sagging epidermis (elevates and tightens your skin layer).

- Aids in removing dark circles round the eyes.

- Aids in liberating your skin layer from shaded areas and hyper-pigmentation.

- Brightens the complexion.

- Exceedingly increases the curing period of breakouts and acne. Helping these epidermis issues overall.

- Has the capability to heal and relieve rosacea.

- Supports product penetration.

- Goodies TMJ disorder and migraines.

- It's an alternative solution to shots and face-lift surgery (when used frequently in the home or when obtaining treatments from a qualified practitioner).

How will You Select a Gua-sha Tool?

Gua-sha tools can be found in different designs, sizes and forms. Some devices are created from pet bone and horn, some from gemstones (like jade or increased quartz). Several professionals utilize the Chinese soup spoons. I've even seen the cover of the cup jar (one with curved and soft sides) within a pinch being used.

Trending at this time is usually *quartz and jade*.

Jade establishes an atmosphere for inviting serenity and purity as well as promoting fertility, balance and deep recovery.

Rose quartz *establishes and aids in restoring tranquillity deep into the heart. It is the stone of universal love and promotes unconditional care and compassion.*

Choosing your gua-sha rock is related to choosing a crystal or gemstone. When you can select it out personally (please do that). Choose it up, experience it, observe its feel in your hands. See which catches your attention – if the foremost is sparkling a little more for you personally than others, prefer it!

What's the Main Element to a Rewarding Practice?

Regularity may be the key to maintain a flourishing and sound body. We regularly nourish ourselves with normal water, rest, balanced meals and motion. Likewise, constant gua-sha therapy will prove to be worthwhile. The body doesn't thrive if we are oscillating to either extreme - the guts is always best suited.

Since you will find 20 liters of liquid that circulate through the body each day (and around three liters from the fluid becomes lymph liquid), it is rather supportive to the body to introduce this practice into the daily routine. However, incorporating gua-sha into every day life could be challenging, but carving out a fantastic short amount of time a few days ,weekly, is active (even if it's only two minutes). You might notice the body starting to crave these occasions of self-care.

Pressure and purpose will also be essential to your practice, the touch ought to be very soft as you'll test out different degrees of pressure. But always sweep the gua-sha rock across your face in specific movements. The lighter the touch, the bigger you are assisting the lymph liquid and with a rise of pressure, know you're engaging in muscle. Please be cautious that you should not bruise or cause distress.

How will You Prep Your Skin Layer?

Using a clean face and clean hands, most importantly having a hydrosol *(I love True Botanicals Renew Nutrient Mist, OSEA's Sea Vitamin Boost or Heritage Store's Rose Water)*, then apply facial oil *(I love True Botanicals Renew Radiance Oil, OSEA's Undaria Argan Oil or Shiva Rose face oil)* around see your face and neck using the fundamental oil left on the hands, grease up your gua-sha tool. Then start – all the while taking deep cleansing breaths.

How will You Perform Gua-sha?

Cleanse Face and Hands - After blow drying the facial skin using a clean washcloth, generously mist your face. The hydrosol is a superb way to use the fundamental oil - which you'll apply next - deep in to the epidermis, especially towards the layers that want nourishment and hydration. (Suggestion: I only use my washcloth once and it switches into the hamper. When you have issues with breakouts, it's best never to reuse cosmetic towels before cleaning. Bacteria can transferred again to your skin.)

Apply Facial - Gas (from 4-10 drops) on the facial skin and throat, apply gas starting with the forehead and moving down in the direction of draining lymph liquid. This activates motion in epidermis and cells and it's an excellent prep prior to the gua-sha.

Warm Gua-sha tool slightly by rubbing it between your hands. This also greases the tool up slightly such that it doesn't draw on your skin layer in the areas that didn't receive much gas.

Sweep up your guitar neck on both edges - Sweep very

softly over your Adam's apple, that is even more of an instant sweep to activate your REN collection. (The REN route in Chinese medication collects the body's yin energy, guards the problems from the stomach, chest, neck, mind and face.)

Sweep under your chin - from your guts away to your earlobe, keeping your tool smooth. If you like, support the epidermis under your chin together with your additional thumb as you glide these devices back to your earlobes in the contrary direction.

Sweep from the centre of the chin over your jawline - again toward your earlobes, you are able to gently jiggle the ears to encourage the liquid to drain down the throat towards the lymph nodes in the bottom, just above your collarbone.

Sweep underneath your cheekbone – Pick up significant amounts of liquid that's commonly stored here and direct it toward your hairline. You are able to slightly and lightly jiggle your tool on the hairline.

Sweep over your cheekbones - finishing in the hairline.

Very gently sweep under your eye - I love sweeping

through the area of the attention relocating toward the midline, the muscle agreement with this path as well as the lymph offers little streams moving down from the attention entirely from the inner corner from the focus on the outer part. But if it appears better to sweep from the inside edge from the care towards the hairline - that is an even more traditional path for gua-sha.

Sweep around the eyebrow out toward the hairline or even more from your own brow bone - (in the forehead) finishing on the hairline; when you sweep up, take action in tiny areas, moving along the eyebrow in three to five 5 sections.

Sweep from the middle of your eyebrows over another eye or even more towards the hairline - Detect in any case should your clairvoyance seems to be more activated.

Sweep through the centre from the forehead out to the hairline - Among the best techniques hails from Britta Plug of Britta Beauty in NYC. She sweeps from the guts from the forehead and doesn't touch the hairline and proceeds into the locks, behind the ears and down the throat. (It feels divine).

Now caress the other part of your face - starting again together with your neck and working through the steps.

Glide down the medial side - When you've completed the other part of your face, finish the task by sweeping down the throat to assist with enduring drainage. Carefully keep the tool toned and placed underneath your jawbone, gently sweep down the throat towards the collarbone.

Essential ideas to help you practice:

- I would recommend sweeping each area at minimal 3x for extended practice, sweep up to 10 times.

- Maintain your tool level to your skin layer (about 15 degrees) instead of getting the benefit of the tool at 90 degrees to your skin layer.

- Whenever your tool begins to pull or draw on your skin layer, apply a bit more gas for an improved slide.

- Have fun trying out which aspect and type of tool best suits your face. Remember, what feels correct for you personally may appear unique from how it's seen in videos.

How often Should I Practice Gua-sha?

I would suggest incorporating gua-sha into the self-care program daily, however when it begins to feel like an activity, have a rest.

Precisely what does it Feel like?

Gua-sha is known to be very relaxing, mainly when the pressure is right, using adoring and mild strokes be intentional with your touch. It'll feel just like you are sweeping the gua-sha on the stunning, soft skin of an infant.

You may feel the fluids moving, which is fantastic! You may feel your skin layer coming alive or as if it's returning and waking up. I often start the medication in the still left, since it is reported to be the medial side of the feminine energy, which is more utilized at receiving. I've remarked that when the rest of the body gets it, it primes the most responsive part of the body.

How excessive could Gua-sha be?

Avoid gua-sha if you have recently received injections. Botox requires at least staying for a fortnight.

Avoid gua-sha over cystic acne, pimples and start lesions since it is only going to irritate contaminated areas, but gua-sha is quite beneficial inside the breakout. Draining below the breakout allows the lymph to move poisons towards the lymph nodes.

Repeat each heart stroke inside the same region, only ten times. If you're repeating the sweep way too much, you might cause an excessive amount of activation. Liquids are potent, you could finish off moving an excessive amount of spleen at a time, causing detoxification symptoms (for example dizziness or emotions of decrease using the flu).

Chapter 9

Cellulite

Cellulite usually starts around the hips and thighs and mostly along the yang meridians, the place to start is usually the Gall Bladder. Small yang meridian, the **Qi** in the Gall Bladder is usually less than in the other yang meridians. Cellulite explains the dimpling of your skin layer, triggered from the protrusion of subcutaneous extra fat in to the dermis, creating an undulating junction in the middle of your epidermis and subcutaneous adipose cells.

The Spleen nourishes muscle and fat, the function of the Spleen is to distribute fat evenly through the body, especially in the periphery. Regarding cellulite, the excess fat distribution is affected and fat seems to stagnate without circulation in a few regions of your body. So, on one hand, there is without a doubt excess fat and also there is without a doubt that it is as a result of poor circulation. This creates the picture of imbalance explained above.

However, we likewise have the problem in the meridian along which this problem occur - that may be Gall

Bladder but it may also be Urinary Bladder and even Stomach, depending on the patient. So both Spleen as well as the affected meridians needs to be well balanced.

Body Acupuncture Treatment

Example - cellulite around the lateral a part of thighs

- Gall Bladder - UB 19 (Back-Shu stage), GB 37 (Luo level).

- Spleen - UB 20 (Back-Shu period), St 40 (Luo place).

- Local needles and moving cup massage.

- Two sessions weekly, 8-10 sessions altogether.

This treatment principle can be employed by Atlanta divorce attorneys affected by meridian. For example, for the Bladder meridian - you should use UB 28 (the Back-Shu position, to improve the function) and UB 58 (the Luo-connecting point of yang meridian, to tonify the yang and reduce the yin aspect).

Local treatment is fairly useful if well performed.

Patients sometimes want to hurry through the neighborhood process because cupping massage therapy isn't so pleasant - it's necessary to be patient while taking this treatment.

Special Local Therapy

If the affected area is along the Gall Bladder meridian, this treatment ought to be achieved in two halves, with the average person lying using one side 1st and having all of the tiny needles and cupping and then going through the other aspect and obtaining the same treatment.

- Lying privately factors on your own body - UB 18, UB 20, St 40, GB 37.

- At exactly the same time, about 10 to 15 local tiny needles around the cellulite (15-20 cm tiny needles of 0.20 mm gauge) are inserted wholly and perpendicularly, at about 3 cm distance in one another.

- Both body needles and local needles are left in the body for 20 minutes.

- After all the needles have been removed, apply St

John's wort oil sparingly on the spot of cellulite. Usually, do not overdo this as it'll reduce friction for the massage therapy.

- Place a large cup (for a specific cellulite glass) at the reduced end from the thigh using an open fire for creating vacuum pressure and slip the container along the spot before epidermis becomes red. This technique is fairly unpleasant for the average person, and if very sore your vacuum could possibly be reduced. The massage therapy takes a minute.

- The person may remark that his legs feels very light following a treatment.

- Treatment is administered twice regularly, about 8-10 times like a course.

What can an Average Person do at Home?

As cellulite is stagnation of fat, the average person can do quite a number of at home in order to avoid its formation and to improve circulation.

- Foods that creates fat tissue in the body are; fatty foods, fatty dairy food (low-fat dairy food should be consumed in smaller amounts), processed sugars, and sugar (though wholemeal, fruits, sugars, and honey are fine). These food types ought to be prevented.

- When fat tissue becomes too thick, the blood flow is affected. It is therefore crucial that the average person drinks clean water regularly and stay hyderated the whole day - the regularity is more important compared to the number consumed. Hot water surpasses cool, which is impressive and surmounts to how quickly patients enjoy hot water.

- Finally, there is a need to work daily around the cellulite, massaging it with very soft spiky toners and pummelling these areas to break the stagnation. Seated cross-legged on the floor and moving sideways and ahead and back in this position, results in friction on parts of cellulite (bum walking), for quarter-hour every day in the comfort of the home is definitely an additional solution to greatly help improve blood flow.

Gua-sha Massage Therapy Cellulite Singapore

Seeking a cure for the unequal, lumpy epidermis on your hips, thighs or buttocks? The Gua-sha Massage therapy Cellulite brings you everything you need. You no longer need to be ashamed of your own physical appearance.

Meet Gua-Sha: The Cellulite Remover

Gua-Sha massage therapy is a therapy technique used to deal with several ailments, these includes: pains and aches, strains, lumbar stress, arthritis rheumatoid and heat heart stroke. The activation of blood flow triggers its therapeutic impact and this relieves bloodstream stagnation.

Moreover, the Gua-sha Massage Cellulite eliminates or reduces the introduction of cellulite in the body.

Advantages of Gua-Sha:

- Improves hydration levels.

- Relieves stress.

- Eliminates or reduces Cellulite.

- Relaxes face muscles.

- Improves blood flow etc.

Gua-sha Massage Therapy treatment:

If your skin layer is oily and a Gua-Sha device is gently utilized to scrape over the top of the affected area, this promotes breakage of surface adhesion, increases circulation and enhances lymph drainage and firmness. In addition, it solves the issues of fats cells and encourages a smoother appearance.

Gua-Sha can be done on any part of the body. It may be performed on Atlanta divorce attorney's part of the body, even with the facial skin. It can help to relax your skin layer and improve blood flow in the facial skin as well as improve collagen creation, it makes your skin layer look more radiant and reduces lines and wrinkles.

Also, people utilize massage techniques or dry brushing to remove cellulite. The triggering of cells manually really helps to improve blood flow and in addition reduces disposed tissues, specifically in keeping energies like unwanted weight. Thus, it boosts skin radiance.

CPSIA information can be obtained
at www.ICGtesting.com
Printed in the USA
BVHW042124100821
614102BV00014B/256